Unleashing Al Superpowers

Deciphering Personal Growth and Self-Discovery
Methods for Resilient Parenting with ADHD Children

Michele L. Valdez

Introducing the exclusive and captivating world of *Michele L. Valdez.* Immerse yourself in the timeless elegance and creativity that defines our brand. Experience the unparalleled craftsmanship and attention to detail that sets us apart. Discover the essence of sophistication and style with our exquisite collection.

Table of Contents

Preface

Are you prepared to change the way you view ADHD—from a handicap to an advantage? Are you sick and weary of hearing what your ADHD prevents you from doing?

Greetings from a revolutionary path of self-realization and strength. Through "Unleashing ADHD Superpowers," we extend an invitation to accept your individual cognitive style and discover your hidden potential. A world where neurodiversity is valued as a vital asset has replaced antiquated ideas of ADHD as a handicap.

It's time to change the story. Embark on an empowering journey where your distinct cognitive style is not a barrier to overcome but rather a powerhouse just waiting to be unlocked. In "Unleashing ADHD Superpowers," the conventional wisdom on ADHD is reversed.

By redefining common features like hyperactivity, impulsivity, and distractibility as beneficial assets rather than constraints, we question the conventional thinking around ADHD. We dispel myths and preconceptions by utilizing the most recent findings in psychology and neuroscience, giving you the confidence to proudly accept your neurodivergent identity.

There are unique difficulties associated with having ADHD, but don't worry—we've got you covered. We offer practical methods in this guide for handling typical symptoms of ADHD, ranging from organizing and time management to impulse control and emotional regulation. You'll discover useful advice and methods to support you in thriving, regardless of whether you're having trouble focusing or are feeling overstimulated by your surroundings.

Uncover Your ADHD Brain's Hidden Strengths

Your ADHD traits—from hyperfocus to unconventional thinking—are more than simply quirky characteristics; they hold the secret to realizing your greatest potential. With captivating stories, useful activities, and knowledgeable advice, this book will teach you how to use your neurodiversity to your advantage and succeed in all facets of life.

Convert Obstacles into Opportunities

Bid farewell to feeling confused and overpowered. With "Unleashing ADHD Superpowers," you'll discover how to take daily challenges head-on, use setbacks as stepping stones, and accept your ADHD as a strength rather than a source of guilt.

What You Stand to Gain:

Empowerment: As you accept your neurodivergent identity, rediscover your feeling of pride and purpose.

Useful Techniques: Discover doable methods for enhancing self-control, organization, and attention in many facets of your life.

Community: Make connections with like-minded people and become a part of a welcoming community that celebrates neurodiversity.

Take Part in the Movement

It's time to accept the full potential of your ADHD brain and let go of outmoded labels. Are you prepared to redefine success and unleash your superpowers? Get your copy of "Unleashing ADHD Superpowers" in advance to start your journey of self-awareness and change. The beginning of your future is today.

Introduction

Discover the ultimate solution to banish overwhelm and gain confidence in supporting your child with ADHD like never before! Are you yearning for expert advice and compassionate assistance to effortlessly navigate the intricate journey of raising a neurodivergent child?

Introducing "Unleashing ADHD Superpowers" – an extraordinary solution meticulously crafted to empower parents just like you. Discover a groundbreaking toolkit filled with powerful strategies, invaluable tools, and unwavering support, all tailored to help you thrive on your remarkable ADHD parenting journey.

Discover the Power of "Unleashing ADHD Superpowers"

Experience the power of a holistic approach.

At our organization, we recognize that raising a child with ADHD goes beyond simply addressing symptoms. It's about cultivating resilience, boosting self-esteem, and nurturing your child's exceptional strengths. Experience a parenting approach that goes above and beyond mere behavior management techniques. Our method takes into account the emotional, relational, and academic aspects of ADHD parenting, providing a comprehensive and sustainable support system for your family.

Discover the Power of Practical Strategies!

Experience the end of uncertainty and annoyance! Discover the incredible power of "Unleashing ADHD Superpowers"! This comprehensive guide provides you with a wealth of evidence-based strategies and actionable tips that are specifically tailored to meet your child's unique needs and challenges. Say goodbye to frustration and hello to success as you unlock the full potential of your child's ADHD superpowers! Discover the power of our proven techniques that will empower you to navigate every aspect of ADHD parenting with confidence and competence. From creating effective routines to enhancing communication skills and advocating for your child's education, we have the tools you need to succeed.

Experience the power of community support.

Discover the comfort of knowing that you are never alone on this incredible journey. Experience the power of connection and support by joining our vibrant community of parents, experts, and individuals who understand the challenges and triumphs of ADHD firsthand. Discover a place where you can find understanding, guidance, and a sense of belonging. Join us today and be a part of a community that truly cares. Experience the power of community as you celebrate your triumphs, discover invaluable guidance, and discover comfort in the knowledge that you belong to a caring and empathetic network committed to fostering growth and prosperity for all.

Unlock your full potential with our Personal Growth program. Discover new skills, develop your strengths, and achieve personal success like never before. Embrace the journey of self-improvement and watch yourself grow into the

Discover the incredible potential of ADHD Superpowers, not only for your child but also for yourself. Embrace the journey of empowerment and self-discovery. Embark on a transformative journey of personal growth, resilience, and self-discovery with the power of reflective exercises, mindfulness practices, and self-care strategies. Experience the profound impact of these powerful tools as you unlock your true potential and embrace a life of fulfillment and purpose. Experience a transformative journey as you rediscover the incredible strengths within you, reignite the fire of your passions, and reclaim the pure joy that comes with navigating the challenges of ADHD parenting. Embrace a life filled with grace and authenticity, as you confidently navigate the ups and downs of this unique journey.

Embark on an Exciting Journey Towards a Radiant Future Today!

Discover the key to unlocking your child's full potential and ensuring that ADHD doesn't define their future. Empower them with the support and guidance they truly deserve. Experience the life-changing power of "Unleashing ADHD Superpowers" and unlock a world of transformation, connection, and endless possibilities. Don't wait, order now and begin your extraordinary journey today.

Unlock the potential of holistic ADHD parenting with your very own copy of this book. Experience the transformative power that every child deserves to shine with. Don't miss out!

Chapter 1

Discover the fascinating world of ADHD!

Discover the remarkable world of Attention Deficit Disorder (ADHD and ADD), a captivating brain disorder that impacts an astounding eleven percent of children and an impressive five percent of adults in the United States. Experience the telltale signs of ADHD: a world of distractions, a struggle to focus, a constant battle against time, impulsive decisions that leave you questioning, emotions that run wild, moments of intense concentration, an unstoppable energy, and a professional life that feels out of sync. Discover a world of diverse symptoms, each unique to the different types of ADHD: the focused and introspective inattentive ADHD, the energetic and spontaneous hyperactive or impulsive ADHD, or the dynamic combination of both in combined ADHD.

Discover the groundbreaking findings from neuroscience, brain imaging, and clinical research that challenge the traditional perception of ADHD as a mere behavior disorder. According to the esteemed Thomas E.

DARKISH, Ph.D., Associate Director of the Yale Hospital for Attention and Related Disorders, it's time to rethink our understanding of ADHD. Discover the fascinating truth: ADHD is not just a simple condition, but a remarkable developmental impairment that affects the brain's intricate management system.

Discover the fascinating insights of Joel Nigg, Ph.D., esteemed professor of Psychiatry at Oregon Health & Technology University. According to Dr. Nigg, ADHD is not simply a breakdown of your brain in one solitary location. It is a profound breakdown in the intricate bond, the vital communication systems, and the immaturity within these systems. Uncover the complexities of ADHD and gain a deeper understanding of its impact. Discover the intricate web of interconnections within the brain, where systems seamlessly intertwine through the powerful forces of feelings, attention, behavior, and arousal. Discover the challenges faced by individuals with ADHD - a condition that affects self-control, attention span, and ultimately leads to concentration and psychological difficulties.

Discover why many experts argue that the term "Attention deficit" may be misleading Introducing "Attention Deregulation" - a term that truly captures the essence of ADHD. You see, individuals with ADHD often receive ample attention, but the challenge lies in their ability to direct and sustain it. Imagine a scenario where you require someone's undivided focus, only to find that their attention is scattered. This is precisely what happens to those with ADHD. They may hyper-focus on a task, losing all sense of time, or unintentionally reveal their deepest secrets or thoughts when their concentration wavers. It's a fascinating phenomenon, don't you think?

Unveiling the Secrets: Unraveling the Factors Behind ADHD

Discover the groundbreaking findings of ADHD research, unveiling the undeniable influence of genetics and heredity in distinguishing those who possess the remarkable qualities of ADHD from those who do not. Discover the fascinating world of genetic research as scientists delve into the intricate workings of specific genes. With a particular focus on the neurotransmitter dopamine, these brilliant minds are uncovering potential links to the development of ADHD. Prepare to be amazed by the groundbreaking discoveries that lie ahead. Discover the fascinating findings that reveal how contact with poisons and chemicals can potentially heighten a child's susceptibility to ADHD.

Discover the truth about ADHD - a brain-based genetic disorder that has nothing to do with bad parenting, sugary indulgences, or excessive video game play. Rest assured, the root cause of ADHD lies within the intricate workings of the brain. Discover the fascinating world of ADHD through cutting-edge brain imaging studies and groundbreaking research, which unveil a myriad of physiological variations in the brains of individuals with this condition.

Discover the fascinating findings that indicate children with ADHD are an astounding four times more likely to have inherited this condition from a family member. This compelling evidence strongly suggests a clear hereditary link. Discover the cutting-edge efforts of experts in the United States and Europe as they tirelessly strive to unravel the intricate web of genes that contribute to an individual's vulnerability to ADHD. Discover the groundbreaking research conducted on a multitude of genes, with a special focus on the neurotransmitter dopamine. Uncover the pivotal role this neurotransmitter plays in the development of ADHD. Discover the fascinating world of ADHD, a disorder that is undoubtedly significant. Experts believe that this captivating condition involves not just one, but at least two genes. Uncover the intricate genetic puzzle behind ADHD and delve into the complexities of this remarkable disorder.

Discover the astonishing findings of medical research that reveal a compelling link between hazardous chemicals and our well-being. Uncover the hidden dangers lurking in everyday items like foods, carpeting, flooring, cleaning products, and personal belongings. These seemingly harmless elements may actually be playing a role in the development of disorders such as

ADHD, autism, and learning disabilities. Prepare to be enlightened by the eye-opening connection that science has uncovered. Discover the alarming impact of toxins on brain development, leading to the occurrence of disabilities such as ADHD.

Discover the Three Types of ADHD!

Introducing the remarkable world of ADHD, where you will encounter not just one, not two, but three extraordinary types:

- Introducing the Hyperactive-Impulsive Type - the epitome of energy and spontaneity.

- Introducing the Inattentive Type, formerly known as ADD.

- Introducing the incredible Combined Type!

Experience the unstoppable energy of individuals with the hyperactive-impulsive type of ADHD. They live life in the fast lane, driven by an internal engine that propels them forward. With their boundless enthusiasm, they may find it challenging to resist impulses, resulting in constant movement, fidgeting, and speaking out, even in the most unexpected moments. Discover the thrilling world of individuals who exude spontaneity, a burning desire for immediate results, and an irresistible urge to interject their thoughts.

Discover the remarkable characteristics of individuals with the inattentive type of ADHD, where their attention may wander and their memory may falter. Introducing the whimsical daydreamers who effortlessly lose track of their homework, cell phones, and even the conversations they're engaged in. Discover the remarkable individuals who possess a diverse range of all the symptoms outlined above - the ones with combined-type ADHD.

Unlocking the unique manifestations of ADHD in each individual. Discover the early signs of ADHD that often emerge during the school years. Watch as your child's focus wavers, assignments slip from their mind, and behavior challenges arise, all in an effort to capture the teacher's attention. Discover the remarkable trend: adult women are now the fastest growing segment receiving

ADHD diagnoses.

Discover a world where symptoms like mood swings, dizziness, and stress are transformed into a clear understanding of ADHD. Experience the power of knowledge as a mother uncovers her own ADHD status through the lens of her child's symptoms. Embrace the journey of self-discovery and find empowerment in understanding.

Discover the Telltale Signs of ADHD

Discover the power of accurate ADHD diagnosis with the help of the fifth edition of the renowned Diagnostic and Statistical Manual of Mental Disorders (DSM-V). Trust the expertise of doctors who utilize these detailed requirements to ensure precise identification. Introducing the remarkable world of ADHD! In the captivating realm of ADHD, the prestigious DSM-V has meticulously curated a list of not one, not two, but nine awe-inspiring symptoms that are indicative of ADHD-Primarily Inattentive. And that's not all! Brace yourself for the exhilarating ADHD-Primarily Hyperactive/Impulsive, which also boasts a magnificent nine symptoms that will leave you in awe. Prepare to be amazed!

Discover the possibility of your child having ADHD, a condition that affects millions of children worldwide. By identifying at least six out of the nine symptoms on our comprehensive list, and observing these symptoms for a minimum of six months, you can gain valuable insights into your child's behavior at home and in school. Don't let ADHD hinder your child's growth and development any longer. Take action now. Discover the telltale signs of these symptoms, all of which must be recognized before the age of twelve. Discover the remarkable fact that older teenagers and adults possess the ability to showcase their uniqueness by demonstrating a mere five of the symptoms.

Introducing the ADHD - Primarily Inattentive Type

Introducing a tendency to occasionally overlook details or make careless errors, whether it be in the realm of academics, professional endeavors, or other activities. This may manifest as a failure to notice or acknowledge important specifics, or a subpar execution of tasks.

Introducing the ultimate solution for those who struggle with concentration! Say goodbye to distractions and hello to laser-like focus. Whether it's during lectures, conversations, or even when reading, our product will help you stay locked in and fully engaged. No more wandering thoughts or lost productivity. Get ready to conquer any task with ease!

Introducing a common occurrence among individuals with disorder: a tendency to become easily distracted, seemingly lost in their own thoughts, and unintentionally disregarding conversations directed towards them.

Introducing a common challenge: a tendency to stray from instructions and leave tasks unfinished. Whether it's schoolwork, assignments, or work responsibilities, they may start with enthusiasm but struggle to maintain focus, easily succumbing to distractions.

Introducing a unique individual who possesses a distinctive flair for creativity and innovation. This individual may occasionally encounter challenges when it comes to organizing tasks and activities. From managing sequential instructions to keeping belongings in order, they may exhibit a touch of untidiness. However, their work remains unparalleled, even in the face of disorganization. While they may struggle with time management and meeting deadlines, their exceptional talents shine through.

Introducing a revolutionary approach to productivity - our solution allows you to effortlessly steer clear of mentally challenging activities. Say goodbye to the stress and strain of engaging your brain, and say hello to a more relaxed and carefree lifestyle. Introducing a versatile tool for all your needs, whether it's tackling schoolwork or conducting research. Perfect for teenagers and adults alike, it excels at planning reviews, completing forms, and even reviewing lengthy documents. Say goodbye to tedious tasks and hello to efficiency!

Introducing a revolutionary solution to end the frustration of misplaced items. Say goodbye to the days of searching for your school materials, pencils, books, tools, wallets, tips, paperwork, eyeglasses, and even your precious mobile phone. With our innovative system, you'll never lose your essentials again.

Introducing a common challenge: the constant battle against unnecessary thoughts. Whether you're a teenager or an adult, it's all too easy to get caught up in unrelated distractions.

Never miss a beat with our revolutionary solution! Say goodbye to forgetfulness when it comes to daily activities. Whether it's performing tasks, running errands, returning calls, paying bills, or keeping appointments, we've got you covered. Stay on top of your game and never let anything slip through the cracks again.

Introducing ADHD - Primarily Hyperactive-Impulsive Type: Unleash your potential!

Experience the dynamic energy of constant movement with our innovative chair design. Say goodbye to sitting still and embrace the freedom to fidget and squirm to your heart's content. Our chair is specially crafted to accommodate your restless nature, allowing you to stay engaged and focused throughout the day.

Introducing a dynamic individual who refuses to conform to the norm. They possess an irresistible urge to rise when others remain seated. Prepare to be captivated by their unyielding spirit.

Are you tired of your little ones constantly running around or climbing in places where it's not appropriate? Say goodbye to those endless moments of frustration and hello to a more peaceful environment.

Experience the undeniable sensation of restlessness, whether you're a child or an adult.

Introducing the ultimate advocate for personal space and privacy.

Experience the thrill of being constantly on the move, always full of vibrant energy and never tied down to one place. They are the ones who are always "away from home," living life to the fullest. Introducing a revolutionary solution for those who struggle with restlessness and find it challenging to maintain composure in various settings, such as restaurants or conferences. Say goodbye to the constant battle of keeping up with the demands of everyday life. Discover a new level of tranquility and ease with our groundbreaking product.

Engage in captivating conversations.

Experience the thrill of jumping into people's conversations and effortlessly completing their phrases. Become the ultimate conversationalist and leave a lasting impression.

Introducing an individual who simply despises change or enduring lengthy queues. Waiting in line? Not their cup of tea.

Introducing a remarkable individual who possesses a unique ability to captivate attention and make their presence known. This extraordinary individual may occasionally find themselves unable to resist the urge to interject or encroach upon the lives of others. Whether it's enthusiastically joining conversations, immersing themselves in video games or activities, or even borrowing items without prior consent, this individual has an undeniable knack for making their mark. They possess an innate desire to be at the forefront of what others are doing, sometimes even attempting to exert their influence and take control. Truly a force to be reckoned with!

Discover the process of diagnosing ADHD.

Discover the power of an ADHD test, designed to uncover the telltale signs of attention deficit hyperactivity disorder. Discover the fascinating world of ADHD, a condition that unveils three distinct sub-types, each with its own captivating characteristics. Dive into the spectrum of intensity, where signs emerge in a mesmerizing array of variations. Explore the intricate web of comorbid conditions that intertwine with ADHD, adding complexity to the analysis and treatment process. Brace yourself for a journey of discovery like no other.

Discover the intricate process of diagnosing ADHD, where meticulous test-taking and thorough evaluation are the key components. Discover the first step towards understanding ADHD with a visit to the doctor, but brace yourself for an enlightening journey that goes far beyond.

Discover the surprising truth: the vast majority of doctors lack the specialized training needed to accurately diagnose ADHD and recognize its telltale symptoms. Discover the elite few who possess the specialized training required to execute the meticulous and comprehensive evaluation that is essential.

Discover the true value of an ADHD diagnosis, carefully evaluated against the comprehensive criteria outlined in the esteemed DSM-V. Discover the power of diagnosis as it delves into the patient's comprehensive medical record. Accompanied by cutting-edge neuropsychological screening, this process uncovers invaluable insights into their unique strengths and weaknesses. Furthermore, it aids in the identification of any comorbid or related conditions, ensuring a thorough understanding of the patient's overall health.

Discover the fascinating truth that many doctors have uncovered: the hidden world of ADHD symptoms that lay dormant until later in life. Brace yourself for a revelation that will leave you astounded. Yes, it's true - this phenomenon primarily affects individuals with the inattentive type of ADHD. Prepare to have your mind blown!

Unlocking the mysteries of an adult's diagnosis requires a touch of finesse that surpasses the simplicity of diagnosing a child. Introducing the revolutionary DSM-V sign guide - your ultimate resource for diagnosing adults! Say goodbye to outdated methods that focus solely on children. Our meticulously crafted steps are specifically designed to cater to the unique needs of adults. Discover a new level of accuracy and effectiveness with the DSM-V sign guide for adults. Discover the meticulous and scientific process of diagnosing ADHD in adults, expertly conducted by a dedicated ADHD specialist who takes the time to conduct a thorough evaluation.

"Discover the groundbreaking DSM-V requirements, meticulously crafted through extensive research, specifically tailored for children aged four to seventeen," declares DARKISH, the esteemed assistant clinical professor of psychiatry at the prestigious Yale College and University School of Medication. Experience the incredible outcome that leads most clinicians to effortlessly loosen their standards when it comes to age. Discover the fascinating findings of recent research, which suggest that for certain individuals, symptoms may not become apparent until adolescence. It is during this crucial stage of development that self-management challenges begin to emerge, shedding light on the importance of early detection and intervention. Discover how doctors can diagnose adults with just 4 or 5 critical symptoms.

Discover the Ultimate Solution for Managing ADHD Symptoms

Discover the unparalleled effectiveness of stimulants as the premier treatment option for ADHD. Extensive studies have unequivocally demonstrated their unmatched reliability in addressing this condition. "Discover the undeniable power of medication for managing ADHD," declares Russell A. Barkley, Ph.D., esteemed Medical teacher of psychiatry and pediatrics at the prestigious Medical School of SC. When adults inquire about the necessity of using drugs to regulate their ADHD, Dr. Barkley's response is refreshingly straightforward: Medication works." Discover the transformative power of the perfect medication and witness a remarkable improvement in your ADHD symptoms.

Introducing the groundbreaking clinical practice guidelines crafted by the esteemed American Academy of Child and Adolescent Psychiatry (AACAP). These guidelines, meticulously curated and backed by a summary of not one, not two, but a staggering seventy-eight studies, have unequivocally declared medication as the premier treatment for ADHD in children. The evidence is resounding, with a resplendent chorus of studies consistently endorsing the use of stimulants as the gold standard in non-drug treatment for ADHD. Trust in the wisdom of the AACAP and embark on a transformative journey towards optimal care for your child.

Introducing the groundbreaking Multi-Modal MTA Cooperative Group Research, a highly acclaimed study that reveals the ultimate solution for ADHD in children.

According to this influential research, combining medication with behavior therapy may just be the perfect treatment. In fact, the study concedes that a pharmacological intervention for ADHD outperforms a behavioural treatment alone. Discover the power of this revolutionary approach today!

Discover the telltale signs of ADHD

Discover the fascinating world of children with ADHD. It's not that they can't pay attention while they're doing things - they simply have a penchant for indulging in their vivid fantasies and daydreams, even while hard at work. However, when faced with repetitive or bothersome tasks, they quickly snap out of their reverie.

Are you struggling to stay focused on one task? If so, you're not alone. Many children with ADHD face this challenge, constantly jumping from one task to another without ever finishing anything. They may even skip important steps along the way. But don't worry, there are solutions to help you overcome this common problem. Discover the art of time management and effortlessly organize school work with ease. Unlock the secret to success that sets these children apart from the rest. Introducing the incredible world of kids with ADHD! These extraordinary individuals possess a unique ability to think outside the box, but sometimes find it challenging to pay attention to the world around them. To unlock their full potential, they thrive in serene and tranquil environments that allow them to fully immerse themselves in their tasks. Discover the power of focus and concentration in these remarkable kids!

Symptoms of Inattention in Children

Experience difficulty concentrating, constantly battling distractions, or losing interest in tasks prematurely.

Introducing our revolutionary product: the unparalleled ability to captivate your attention! Say goodbye to those who seem not to listen when spoken to, and say hello to a world where every word is heard and cherished.

Introducing the solution for those who are tired of forgetfulness and struggling to remember instructions. Say goodbye to the frustration of not being able to concentrate on details and making careless mistakes. Experience a new level of focus and accuracy with our innovative product.

Struggling to stay organized? Finding it challenging to prepare and complete tasks? We've got you covered.

Introducing the all-new, highly efficient Homework and Item Management System! Say goodbye to the days of losing or misplacing your valuable belongings. With our revolutionary technology, you'll never have to worry about missing homework, books, toys, or any other items again. Stay organized and keep everything in its rightful place with ease. Upgrade your life today with our state-of-the-art solution!

Unleash Your Potential: Discover the Link Between Hyperactivity and ADHD

Discover the unmistakable hallmark of ADHD: hyperactivity. Introducing the unstoppable force of nature - children with hyperactive symptoms of attention deficit disorder! While most kids are naturally energetic, these extraordinary individuals take it to a whole new level with their constant movement. Brace yourself for a whirlwind of activity! Experience the thrill of multitasking as they effortlessly navigate through a multitude of activities, seamlessly transitioning from one endeavor to the next. Introducing individuals who simply can't resist the urge to move! Even when prompted to relax and take it easy, they find themselves irresistibly tapping their feet, shaking their lower leg, or rhythmically drumming with their fingers. Their energy is simply contagious!

Symptoms of Hyperactivity in Children

Experience the relentless energy of constantly fidgeting and squirming.

Introducing a revolutionary solution for those who struggle with sitting still, doing things quietly, or finding relaxation. Say goodbye to restlessness and hello to tranquility with our innovative product.

Feeling restless?

Engage in captivating conversations that leave a lasting

impression.

Introducing the all-new tantrum-throwing experience!

Discover the Telltale Signs of ADHD

Introducing the remarkable world of children with impulsive ADHD. These extraordinary individuals possess an unparalleled zest for life, often finding themselves irresistibly drawn to new experiences. Their boundless energy and enthusiasm propel them forward, sometimes without pausing to consider the consequences. Unlike their peers, who may carefully deliberate before taking action, these children embrace the thrill of spontaneity. Yet, it is precisely this unique quality that can present challenges when it comes to self-control. Harnessing their exuberance and helping them navigate the world with thoughtfulness and intention is a journey we embark on together. Introducing a group of individuals who possess a unique ability to captivate attention, these remarkable individuals have been recognized for their knack for sparking lively discussions, occasionally venturing into uncharted territories of personal boundaries. With their uncanny talent for posing thought-provoking inquiries, they have been known to leave a lasting impression, even if it means occasionally treading the line of social etiquette.

Discover the power of tailored guidance for children with ADHD. Traditional instructions like "Be patient" and "Hold on a bit" may fall flat, as these exceptional children often have a unique approach to following directions. Unlock their potential with personalized guidance that speaks their language.

Introducing the remarkable world of children with impulsive symptoms of ADHD! These extraordinary individuals possess an unparalleled ability to experience life's ups and downs with an unparalleled intensity. Prepare to be amazed as they navigate the vast spectrum of emotions, from delightful highs to dramatic lows. Witness their incredible talent for overreacting to even the smallest of things, transforming the ordinary into the extraordinary. Brace yourself for a rollercoaster ride of mood swings, as these exceptional children captivate and astonish with their boundless energy and zest for life.

Witness the transformative power of this phenomenon as it casts a shadow on one's reputation, causing others to perceive them as lacking in respect, eccentric, or even impolite.

Discover the telltale signs of impulsivity in children.

Unleash actions without a second thought.

Introducing the Guess-Maker Extraordinaire! No need to waste precious time on problem-solving when you can simply make educated guesses. And why wait to be called on when you can confidently blurt out answers without even hearing the entire question? Get ready to embrace the thrill of uncertainty!

Discover the art of engaging in lively conversations and captivating games with others.

Discover the art of seamless communication with our expert guidance. Say goodbye to interruptions and hello to perfect timing. Master the art of emotional intelligence and keep your feelings in check. No more outbursts or tantrums. Experience the power of effective communication.

Unlocking the Hidden Impact of ADHD in Children

Unlock your true potential with ADHD - a condition that has no correlation with intelligence or skill. Embrace your unique abilities and soar to new heights! Discover the remarkable positive characteristics that children with attention deficit disorder possess:

Unleash the Power of Creativity: Witness the awe-inspiring potential of children with ADHD as they tap into their boundless imagination. Discover the untapped potential of children who possess the remarkable ability to daydream and juggle ten different thoughts simultaneously. These young minds have the power to transform into exceptional problem solvers, boundless fountains of ideas, and visionary inventive designers. Introducing the extraordinary world of children with ADHD - where distractions become opportunities and hidden gems are revealed. These remarkable individuals possess a unique ability to perceive what others may overlook. Prepare to be amazed by their unparalleled vision.

Unleash the Power of Versatility: Discover how children with ADHD have a unique ability to analyze their choices simultaneously, allowing them to stay open to a world of different ideas and possibilities.

Experience the thrill of constant excitement and endless spontaneity with children who have ADHD. Say goodbye to boredom and hello to a life filled with non-stop adventure! Experience the whirlwind of thoughts and vibrant personalities that captivate their every moment. Discover the undeniable truth: when they're not causing frustration, they become an absolute delight to spend time with.

Unleash the power within: Witness the incredible vigour and unwavering drive of children with ADHD. When they find their motivation, they channel it into their work and play with unparalleled intensity, striving for nothing short of success. Unlocking their focus can be quite the challenge when they're engrossed in a task that truly matters to them, especially if it's an engaging and dynamic experience.

Discover the possibility of ADHD.

Discover the truth about your child's behavior. Just because they show signs of inattention, impulsivity, or hyperactivity, it doesn't automatically mean they have ADHD. Uncover the real story behind their actions. Discover the fascinating world of medical conditions, mental disorders, and stress, all of which can manifest symptoms that may resemble those of ADHD. Unlock the key to understanding ADHD with a comprehensive analysis. Take the first step towards clarity by consulting a skilled mental doctor who can provide a precise diagnosis and expert guidance. Discover the path to overcoming challenges and finding the support you need.

Discover the world of learning disabilities, where challenges become opportunities. Unleash your potential in reading, writing, creative skills, and vocabulary. Embrace the journey of growth and empowerment.

Experience the transformative power of major life events or distressing encounters. Whether it's a relocation, the loss of a loved one, bullying, or a divorce, these moments have the potential to shape us and propel us towards personal growth.

Introducing a range of psychological disorders that can impact your well-being, including anxiety, depression, and bipolar disorder.

Introducing a range of behavioural disorders that can impact individuals' lives. From conduct disorder to reactive attachment disorder and oppositional defiant disorder, these conditions can present unique challenges. Introducing a range of medical conditions that can impact your well-being. From thyroid problems to neurological conditions, epilepsy to sleep issues, we understand the importance of addressing these concerns.

Unlocking the Potential: Assisting a Child with ADHD

Discover the potential underlying cause of your child's symptoms of inattention, hyperactivity, and impulsivity - ADHD. Left untreated, these symptoms can escalate and lead to a multitude of challenges. Discover the secret to unlocking your child's full potential. Say goodbye to academic struggles, frequent trouble, and social challenges. Our revolutionary solution empowers children to concentrate, control themselves, excel in school, and effortlessly make friends. Don't let your child miss out on a bright future. Experience the transformation today! Discover the transformative power of overcoming frustrations, unlocking a world of heightened self-esteem and harmonious relationships with your loved ones. Say goodbye to stress and disagreements, and embrace a life filled with confidence and tranquillity.

Discover how treatment can transform your child's symptoms. Discover the power of seeking professional help if your child is facing challenges with symptoms resembling ADHD. Don't keep it to yourself - take action today! Discover a powerful solution to address your child's symptoms of hyperactivity, inattention, and impulsivity - all without the need for a formal diagnosis of attention deficit disorder. Experience the transformative power of our comprehensive treatment plan. Take the first steps towards a brighter future for your child by enrolling them in therapy. Our team of dedicated professionals will guide them towards growth and healing. Fuel their potential with nourishing, wholesome meals and regular exercise, ensuring their physical and mental well-being. Create a harmonious environment at home by reorganizing and eliminating distractions, allowing your child to focus and thrive. Together, let's embark on this journey towards a happier, healthier life.

Discover the power of taking action when your child receives an ADHD diagnosis. Take the first step by scheduling an appointment with your child's trusted doctor or therapist. Together, you can create a personalized treatment plan that caters to your child's unique needs.

Discover the powerful solution for older children struggling with ADHD: a comprehensive approach that includes behavioural therapy, parent(s) education and training, invaluable interpersonal support, and expert assistance in school. Discover the power of incorporating drugs as part of a comprehensive treatment plan for attention deficit disorder. While drugs are an effective tool, they should always be complemented by other therapeutic approaches.

Discover the Best Parenting Options for Empowering Children with ADHD

Attention, mothers! If your child is bursting with energy, struggling to focus, or constantly on the move, it might be a sign of something more. Yes, we're talking about ADHD - a condition that demands your strength and determination to help your little one listen, complete tasks, and find stillness. Don't ignore the signs!

Experience the convenience of uninterrupted monitoring without the hassle or fatigue. Are you tired of feeling like your child is running the show? Don't worry, because there are simple yet effective strategies you can implement to regain control while nurturing your child's development.

Discover the power of effective parenting strategies that

can make a significant impact in resolving behavioral problems, even though attention deficit disorder is not caused by bad parenting. Unlock the potential of children with ADHD through the power of clear communication, enticing rewards, and heartfelt appreciation for their remarkable behavior. Discover the essential ingredients for a thriving life: love, support, and encouragement. Give yourself and others the gift of these invaluable elements that fuel personal growth and happiness. Discover the multitude of strategies that parents can employ to effectively diminish the telltale signs of ADHD, all while preserving the child's inherent vitality, exuberance, and imagination.

Invest in your well-being to ensure you can provide the best care for your child. Prioritize self-care by nourishing your body with healthy food and staying active through regular exercise. Remember to give yourself ample rest to recharge. Take proactive steps to minimize stress and seek solace in the support of your loved ones, your child's doctor, and their instructors. Your well-being is crucial in creating a nurturing environment for your child.

Empower your child with a firm yet nurturing approach. Guide them towards maintaining focus and organization by diligently completing daily tasks. Streamline their routine to make it more manageable and efficient. Additionally, encourage your child to actively participate in wholesome activities that promote their overall well-being.

Experience the power of clear instructions and simple rules. Discover the magic of knowing exactly what will happen when you follow them or dare to break them. And that's not all - be rewarded with motivation and even a delightful gift every single time. Embrace the art of effective communication and unlock a world of possibilities.

Experience the transformative power of invigorating exercise and restorative sleep. Discover the incredible benefits of exercise for children with ADHD. Experience enhanced focus and accelerated brain development through the power of physical activity. Experience the incredible benefits of our product, which not only enhances focus and attention, but also promotes a restful night's sleep. By improving sleep quality, it has the potential to alleviate the symptoms associated with ADHD. Discover the power of our solution today!

Discover the power of nourishing your child's body with healthy meals to effectively manage the symptoms of ADHD. Introducing the ultimate secret to a healthier lifestyle: meticulously crafted, well-balanced meals or snacks, strategically timed every 3 hours. Say goodbye to the temptations of junk and sweet food as you embark on this transformative journey towards optimal well-being.

Empower your child to cultivate meaningful connections and nurture their active listening skills. Unlock the power of observation by urging him to meticulously observe the subtle nuances of people's expressions and body language. With this heightened awareness, he can effortlessly enhance his interactions and forge deeper connections with others.

Discover the Perfect School Options for Children with ADHD!

Discover the transformative power of learning to solve

ADHD. Unlock your full potential by staying focused and engaged in your surroundings. Say goodbye to distractions and hello to productivity. Don't let your valuable time go to waste. Stay present and absorb information like never before.

Discover the essential expectations set by the school for children: Sit down with intent; Engage in active listening; Harness your concentration; Embrace adherence to instructions; Channel your unwavering focus. Discover the challenges that children with ADHD face, not due to lack of preparation, but because their brilliant minds refuse to comply. Discover the incredible potential of children with ADHD in the classroom!

Discover the multitude of strategies that parents and educators can employ to empower children with ADHD to flourish in the classroom. Unlock the true potential of every child by meticulously analyzing their unique strengths and weaknesses. Through innovative and creative techniques, we empower children to enhance their focus, perseverance, and problem-solving skills. Witness their incredible journey as they explore and unleash their full potential.

Chapter 2

Discover the telltale signs of ADHD!

Introducing our revolutionary solution for children who occasionally find it challenging to capture attention, actively listen, adhere to instructions, maintain composure, or exhibit patience. Introducing a revolutionary solution for children with ADHD. Experience a world where challenges become opportunities and frequent occurrences become manageable.

Discover the telltale signs that may indicate your child has ADHD:

Introducing: The Inattentive Dilemma! For kids who are easily distracted, concentrating their attention and staying focused on a task can be quite the challenge. But fear not, we have the solution! Introducing a group of individuals who possess a unique approach to following instructions. With an uncanny ability to overlook important details and a tendency to leave tasks unfinished, they bring a fresh perspective to any project. Indulge in the art of daydreaming or leisurely dawdling with ample time to spare. Introducing the fascinating world of individuals who possess an uncanny ability to be absent-minded or forgetful, occasionally losing track of even the most important of things.

Introducing Hyperactive: The Ultimate Hyperactive Experience Introducing the vibrant world of children - where energy knows no bounds, curiosity is boundless, and boredom is banished! Introducing a group of individuals who possess an undeniable zest for life, always brimming with energy and enthusiasm. These remarkable individuals may find it challenging to maintain a composed demeanor, as their vibrant spirits simply refuse to be contained. Embrace their vivacious nature as they effortlessly infuse every moment with an electrifying energy that is simply contagious. Experience the thrill of productivity as they race against the clock, only to find that haste can sometimes lead to unfortunate oversights. Experience the thrill as they conquer new heights, defy gravity with daring leaps, and bring chaos to order in the most unexpected ways. Unbeknownst to you, they have the potential to be intrusive and interruptive.

Unleash the power of spontaneity with Impulsive! Designed for kids who dare to act before they think, this innovative product is perfect for those who embrace the thrill of the moment. Say goodbye to hesitation and hello to adventure with Impulsive! Experience the thrill of their spontaneous nature as they fearlessly dive into new adventures, unafraid to disrupt the ordinary. With a boldness that knows no bounds, they seize the moment and embrace the unexpected. Their audacious spirit may lead them to explore uncharted territories, pushing the boundaries of what is deemed possible. Brace yourself for a whirlwind of excitement as they navigate through life with their own unique style. Experience the full spectrum of psychological reactions, intensified to levels beyond what the problem warrants.

Discover the telltale signs of ADHD that vigilant parents and instructors can spot in young children. Discover the truth about children's behavior. It's completely natural for them to be occasionally distracted, restless, impatient, or impulsive. Remember, these common traits do not automatically mean a child has ADHD.

Unlocking the power of focus, productivity, and discipline is a journey that unfolds as a child blossoms. With the invaluable guidance of parents and educators, children embark on a transformative path of acquiring these essential life skills. Discover the secret to engaging children who struggle with sitting still or listening. Discover a world where persistent issues in school, home, and social circles may just be a sign of something bigger - ADHD.

Discover the process of diagnosing ADHD.

Discovering if your child has ADHD is a crucial step towards their well-being. Take the proactive approach and schedule an appointment with your child's trusted doctor today. Experience peace of mind by granting the esteemed doctor the opportunity to meticulously examine your precious child, leaving no stone unturned. From head to toe, the doctor will carefully assess every aspect of your child's body, including the delicate eyes and ears, in order to uncover the underlying cause of the troubling symptoms. Discover the exceptional care of our esteemed doctor, who can expertly guide you towards the perfect solution for your child's needs. With their vast knowledge and experience, they can seamlessly connect you with a highly skilled child psychologist or psychiatrist, ensuring that your child receives the utmost care and support they deserve.

Discovering the truth about ADHD begins with a meticulous examination conducted by skilled doctors. They delve into the depths of a child's health, behavior, and activity, leaving no stone unturned. Engaging in open and meaningful conversations, they skillfully communicate with both parents and children, delving into the symptoms they have astutely observed. Discover how your doctor can help you gain valuable insights into your child's behavior. Be prepared to fill out a comprehensive form that will provide essential information. Plus, don't forget to share a copy with your child's teacher for a collaborative approach to understanding your child's needs.

Discover the power of information gathering as doctors skillfully diagnose ADHD. They carefully assess the situation, taking into account various factors. If a child's distractibility, hyperactivity, or impulsivity surpasses what is considered typical for their age, the doctors are able to identify and diagnose ADHD with precision and accuracy.

Discover the remarkable journey of a child who began showcasing these extraordinary behaviors at a tender age.

Introducing the incredible trio of distractibility, hyperactivity, and impulsivity! These three superpowers have the ability to impact your child's life both at school and at home. Prepare to witness their extraordinary effects!

Introducing a groundbreaking diagnosis that uncovers the true source of the problem, eliminating any doubts about other health or learning challenges.

Discover the remarkable correlation between ADHD and a range of challenges such as learning difficulties, oppositional and defiant actions, and mood and anxiety problems. Fortunately, our dedicated doctors are well-versed in treating these interconnected issues alongside ADHD, ensuring comprehensive care for your child.

Discover the Effective Treatment Options for ADHD!

Discover the transformative power of our comprehensive ADHD treatment options.

- Introducing the revolutionary solution: Medication! Experience the incredible power of activating your brain's natural ability to pay attention, decelerate, and enhance self-control.

- Unlocking Potential: Discover the transformative power of behavior therapy. Our skilled therapists are dedicated to helping children develop essential social, emotional, and organizational skills that may be lacking due to ADHD.

- Unlock the power of parental training: Discover the transformative benefits of equipping parents with the tools to expertly navigate and address behavioral issues that may arise as symptoms of

ADHD.

- Unlocking Academic Success: Discover how dedicated educators can empower children with ADHD to thrive and excel in the classroom.

- Unlock the potential within with the power of the right treatment for ADHD. Discover the power of parental guidance and expert instruction in helping children unlock the secrets to understanding, controlling their attention, behavior, and feelings. Unlock the full potential of your child's development as they journey through the stages of life. Encourage the cultivation of essential skills such as concentration and self-control, empowering them to thrive in an ever-changing world.

- Unlock the potential for success in children by treating ADHD effectively. Experience the potential consequences of this situation: a decrease in self-confidence, the onset of depression, a tendency towards defiance, academic underachievement, engaging in risky behaviors, and potential conflicts within the family unit.

Discover the Ultimate Guide for Parents!

Discover the empowering truth about your child's potential with ADHD:

Get involved: Unlock the secrets of ADHD and expand your knowledge to new heights. Discover the key to unlocking your child's full potential by diligently adhering to the expert guidance and instructions provided by their esteemed doctor. Embrace the transformative power of therapy sessions and ensure you never miss a single one. Your child's journey to success starts with your unwavering commitment.

Discover the perfect dosage: Maximize the effectiveness of your child's ADHD medication by carefully administering the drugs at the precise time and in the correct dosage. Protect your health and safeguard your medicines by storing them in a secure location.

Unlock the power of collaboration with your child's

school: Discover the key to unlocking your child's full potential by inquiring with their esteemed teacher about the possibility of implementing an Individualized Education Programme (IEP). Discover the true potential of your child's academic performance by frequently engaging with her teachers. Unlock the power of communication to empower your child.

Introducing: Parent(s) with Purpose and Warmness! Discover the ultimate parenting techniques to empower your child with ADHD and unlock their full potential. Uncover the strategies that can either enhance or exacerbate ADHD symptoms. Engage in open and supportive conversations with your child about ADHD. Discover the incredible strengths and remarkable qualities of your child.

Experience the power of connection as you join forces with like-minded individuals, fostering a strong support system and raising awareness together. Discover the transformative power of joining a dynamic support group specifically designed for individuals with ADHD. Experience the incredible benefits of enhanced treatment options and gain access to a wealth of invaluable information. Don't miss out on this incredible opportunity to take control of your ADHD journey. Join a support group today!

Empower your child's understanding of ADHD, enlist the expertise of educators and caregivers, and diligently track the strategies that truly make a difference for your child.

Uncover the Intriguing Causes Behind ADHD!

Discover the fascinating mystery behind the brain disorder in ADHD. Discover the undeniable evidence that supports the hereditary nature of ADHD. Discover the fascinating connection between ADHD and genetics. It's not uncommon for children with ADHD to have a family member who also experiences this condition. Could it be that they've inherited it from them? Uncover the intriguing link between ADHD and heredity.

Discover the truth about ADHD: it's not caused by excessive play, poor parenting, or too much sugar.

Unlock the potential for improvement in children with

ADHD through the power of treatment, nourishing their bodies with healthy food, ensuring they receive ample rest and exercise, and providing them with the unwavering support of parents who possess a deep understanding of how to effectively respond to ADHD.

Chapter 3

Discover the 14 undeniable signs of ADHD!

Discover the fascinating world of ADHD!

Introducing the remarkable neurodevelopmental disorder known as Attention Deficit Hyperactivity Disorder (ADHD). This extraordinary condition has the power to impact not only your child's academic performance but also their interpersonal connections. Prepare to witness the profound effects of ADHD on your child's life. Discover the diverse range of symptoms associated with ADHD, making them a challenge to identify.

Discover how the telltale signs of ADHD can be found in every child. Discover the key to diagnosing ADHD with precision and care. Entrust your child's evaluation to a doctor who employs a comprehensive set of criteria.

Discover the fascinating world of ADHD, a condition often identified in children before they reach their teenage years. The average age of diagnosis? A mere seven years old. Discover the telltale signs of ADHD in teenagers. While it's true that these symptoms may have manifested early on, it's crucial to recognize the severity of these indicators.

Discover the 14 telltale signs of ADHD in children!

Discover the power of self-focused behavior!

Discover the telltale sign of ADHD: a remarkable challenge in perceiving and acknowledging the desires and needs of others. Experience the powerful impact of two additional signals: interruption and a noticeable absence of patience.

- The Art of Interruption

    Discover the fascinating world of a child with ADHD, whose self-focused behavior can lead them to interrupt others while they're talking or effortlessly butt into conversations or games they're not part of. Experience the unique perspective of these extraordinary individuals.

- Experience the thrill of anticipation with Trouble

Waiting!

- Discover how children with ADHD can overcome the challenge of waiting their turn during classroom activities or when engaging with peers.

- Experience the rollercoaster of emotions with our latest offering - Emotional Turmoil. Brace yourself for a thrilling journey through love, heartbreak, and everything in between. Let our captivating storytelling and mesmerizing performances

- Discover the challenges faced by a child with ADHD as they navigate the complex world of emotions. Experience the unpredictable nature of their emotions as they unleash anger outbursts at the most unexpected moments, accompanied by fiery temper tantrums.

- Introducing the revolutionary solution to combat fidgeting!

- Introducing the revolutionary solution for children with ADHD who just can't seem to sit still!

Experience the undeniable urge to rise and move, restlessly shifting and wriggling in your seat when all you long for is to unwind and find tranquility.

- Experience the thrill of playing without limits!

- Discover the challenge that fidgeting poses for children with ADHD, hindering their ability to enjoy peaceful and serene playtime or partake in leisurely pursuits.

- Discover the power of completing your to-do list with our revolutionary solution: Unfinished tasks will become a thing of the past. Say goodbye to procrastination and hello to productivity!

- Discover the boundless curiosity of a child with ADHD, as they explore a multitude of interests. Yet, they may encounter challenges when it comes to bringing these passions to fruition. Imagine a world where you have the power to start projects, tasks, or research with ease. However, your curiosity is so insatiable that you often find yourself moving on to the next captivating thing before finishing what you started. Sound familiar?

- Discover the remarkable challenge of paying attention that a child with ADHD may face. Despite someone speaking directly to them, their ability to focus may be hindered, leaving them unable to fully engage. Experience the illusion of being heard and acknowledged, as they assure you of their awareness. Yet, their limitations prevent them from faithfully echoing every word you utter.

- Unlock your full potential by eliminating activities that drain your mental energy. Say goodbye to tasks that leave you feeling exhausted and embrace a life of focus and productivity. Experience the freedom of a clear mind and watch as your efficiency soars to new heights. Take control of your mental energy and unlock a world of endless possibilities.

- Discover the transformative power of focus and attention! Imagine a child who effortlessly engages in activities that demand mental effort, like paying attention in class or completing homework. Say goodbye to distractions and hello to a world of endless possibilities!

Discover the 10 most common mistakes and how to avoid them!

Introducing a challenge that children with ADHD face: they often struggle to follow instructions that involve planning or executing an idea. Experience the possibility of occasional oversights; however, rest assured that it does not imply any lack of effort or intelligence.

Escape into a world of imagination with Daydreaming.

Discover the surprising truth: children with ADHD possess a unique range of qualities that extend far beyond being noisy and loud. Discover yet another telltale sign of ADHD - a condition that affects countless children. Witness how these children, with their unique disposition, often opt for solitude and silence, setting themselves apart from their peers. Introducing the mesmerizing world of a child with ADHD. Watch as they effortlessly drift into their own imaginative realm, leaving the mundane realities behind. Witness their ability to tune out the noise and distractions of the world, as they indulge in the captivating art of daydreaming. Prepare to be amazed as they effortlessly ignore the chaos unfolding around them, lost in their own enchanting universe.

Discover the secret to effortlessly organizing your life with our revolutionary solution: the cure for your inability to put things in order. Say goodbye to chaos and hello to a world of perfect organization.

Introducing the incredible world of a child with ADHD, where keeping up with tasks and monitoring activities becomes an exhilarating challenge. Discover the potential challenges that may arise in the school environment as students navigate the intricate art of balancing research, school assignments, and various other projects.

Introducing: The Revolutionary Solution to Forgetfulness!

Introducing the game-changers: children with ADHD. These incredible young minds possess a unique ability to keep us on our toes. With their captivating forgetfulness, they have the power to surprise us by occasionally forgetting to complete tasks or conduct research. It's like having a live-action adventure unfolding right before your eyes! Introducing a common occurrence: misplacing things. Yes, even playthings are not immune to this phenomenon. It happens to the best of us.

Experience a multitude of symptoms.

Discover the myriad ways in which a child with ADHD showcases its unique symptoms. Imagine the challenge of trying to maintain focus in both the classroom and the comfort of your own home. It's no easy task, but that's exactly what many individuals face.

Discover the Ultimate Solution for Managing Signs of ADHD

Discover the remarkable array of behaviors that every child is bound to exhibit. Unlock the potential of your child's imagination with the power of daydreaming. Embrace their natural curiosity and energy as they fidget and explore the world around them. And don't be alarmed when their enthusiasm leads them to interrupt conversations - it's just a sign of their vibrant and inquisitive mind. Discover the importance of taking the symptoms seriously. It's time to pay attention if your child consistently exhibits signs of ADHD.

Discover how this behavior can have a profound impact on his academic achievements and interpersonal relationships with his closest companions.

Discover the incredible potential for change with our revolutionary ADHD treatment options. Discover the power of collaboration when it comes to your child's ADHD treatment plans. Stay informed and review them together. Experience the peace of mind that comes with taking proactive steps towards your health. Take charge of your well-being by scheduling a meeting with the esteemed doctor, who will guide you on the next course of action. Your health is your greatest asset - don't wait, take action today!

C h a p t e r 4

Discover the Essential Facts about ADHD in Children

Introducing the remarkable Attention Deficit Hyperactivity Disorder, better known as ADHD, a condition that impacts countless children and, in some cases, persists well into adulthood. Unlock the power of analysis at an early age, typically during the preschool years. But don't worry, analysis can still thrive even after your child has outgrown preschool. Discover the challenges that children with ADHD often face - difficulty focusing, coupled with hyperactive and impulsive tendencies. Experience the transformative impact this has on a child's relationships with their family, friends, and teachers.

Discover the growing concern in America surrounding the diagnosis of children with a certain disorder, despite the availability of effective medications for treatment. Discover the undeniable benefits of early medical diagnosis, proven to pave the way for superior treatment options.

Discover the fascinating world of ADHD! Have you ever wondered at what age this captivating condition begins? Brace yourself for the answer: ADHD can actually manifest in infants and toddlers! Yes, you read that right. Even at such a tender age, these little ones can exhibit the symptoms of ADHD. Prepare to be amazed by the early onset of this extraordinary condition! Discover the groundbreaking solutions available for managing ADHD at an early age.

Unlock the potential of your toddler with ADHD! While guidelines for this age group may be scarce, rest assured that there are ways to support and nurture your little one's unique needs. Discover the possibilities and empower your child to thrive!

Discover the latest findings from the prestigious Center for Disease Control and Avoidance (CDC). According to their groundbreaking report, an astounding 6.1 million children between the ages of 2 and 17 in the United States were diagnosed with Attention-

Deficit/Hyperactivity Disorder (ADHD) in 2016. Introducing an astounding collection of data, encompassing a staggering 388,000 children between the ages of 2 and 5 years. Introducing the groundbreaking change that revolutionized the way we approach ADHD diagnosis! Prior to the year 2011, the esteemed American Academy of Pediatrics (AAP) exclusively provided guidelines for identifying this condition in children between the ages of 6 and 12 years old. Brace yourself for the remarkable evolution that lies ahead!

Introducing their groundbreaking guidelines expansion in 2011, they boldly embraced the inclusion of not only preschoolers but also adolescents. This visionary move widened their capacity to cater to the needs of a diverse age group spanning from 4 to 18 years old. Discover the fascinating world of early childhood diagnoses! While some children may receive a diagnosis before the tender age of four, it's important to note that there are currently no established medical guidelines specifically tailored for analyzing this age group. Join us on this journey of understanding and exploration!

Discover the Telltale Signs of Symptoms in Toddlers

Discovering the telltale signs of ADHD in children under the age of four can be quite challenging. Experience the vibrant energy of childhood as your little one embraces their unique journey of growth. Witness the captivating moments of a short attention span, the spontaneous bursts of creativity, the occasional tantrums that reveal their fiery spirit, and the boundless enthusiasm that fuels their every move. These are the hallmark signs of a child's blossoming development, a testament to their vibrant personality and zest for life.

Introducing the incredible abilities of energetic children! These little dynamos, bursting with vitality and enthusiasm, possess an amazing power to focus. And here's the proof: they can effortlessly immerse themselves in captivating stories and meticulously explore the pages of photo books. It's not ADHD, it's just an abundance of energy waiting to be channeled into incredible adventures! Discover the incredible versatility of our products. Not only can they effortlessly tidy up play toys, but they also provide the perfect space to immerse yourself in the joy of solving puzzles. Experience the convenience and satisfaction that our products bring to your everyday life.

Discover how children with ADHD can overcome challenges and accomplish tasks with ease. Prepare to witness a spectacle of unparalleled intensity as they unleash their extreme behavior, causing a whirlwind of disruption to activities and relationships. Discover the key to unlocking the diagnosis of ADHD in children. Witness these remarkable behaviors persisting for a minimum of six months, across various environments including the hallowed halls of academia.

Introducing the energetic world of toddlers with ADHD! Brace yourself for a whirlwind of non-stop action and excitement. These little dynamos are known for their restlessness and their insatiable desire to explore their surroundings. Watch in awe as they run, climb, and conquer anything that comes their way. Get ready to witness the boundless energy and unstoppable spirit of these incredible toddlers!

Unleash the power of your words with non-stop conversation.

Introducing our revolutionary solution for those who struggle to concentrate or pay attention for long. Say goodbye to distractions and hello to enhanced focus with our cutting-edge technology.

Discover the invigorating challenge of staying still, the art of rejuvenating naps, and the joy of savoring meals in a relaxed manner.

Discover the incredible focus of children with ADHD as they immerse themselves in the captivating world of their favorite play toys.

Is your toddler's behavior becoming a bit too much to handle? If you find yourself constantly dealing with intense and frequent outbursts that are impacting your family life, it may be time to seek professional guidance. Don't hesitate to reach out to your child's doctor for a thorough assessment.

Discover the Early Signs of ADHD!

Discover the invaluable tips for diagnosing ADHD, carefully crafted to guide parents and caregivers. Please note that these expert strategies are specifically designed for children aged four and above, ensuring accurate assessments and tailored interventions. Discover the compelling evidence suggesting that doctors are now diagnosing ADHD in children at a younger age.

Discover the compelling factors that could lead a doctor to consider the possibility of ADHD in this particular age group:

- Unlock the secrets of your DNA with the power of genetic factors.

- Discover the potential impact on your child's development if the mother consumed drugs or alcohol during pregnancy.

- Discover the potential risks if the mother smoked during pregnancy.

- Discover the potential impact on your child's health if the mother was exposed to environmental poisons during pregnancy.

- Experience the peace of mind you deserve with our revolutionary solution. Say goodbye to the worries of preterm delivery or low delivery weight. Trust in our innovative approach to ensure a healthy and successful delivery.

- Experience optimal growth with a healthy central nervous system.

- Experience the art of stillness with our revolutionary product. Introducing a delay in movement, conversation, and speech has never been more captivating. Embrace the power of silence and unlock a world of tranquility.

The Solution to Behavioral Difficulties!

Discover the fascinating world of ADHD and its intriguing family background.

Introducing the groundbreaking 2010-2011 Countrywide Report of Children's Health in the U.S.! Prepare to be astounded as we reveal a staggering statistic: an astonishing 194,000 children, aged 2-5, were diagnosed with ADHD during the summer and winter seasons. Brace yourself for the eye-opening findings of this remarkable study!

Discover the Secrets: Unveiling the Art of Diagnosing ADHD by Medical Experts

Discovering ADHD in older children is a crucial step towards helping them thrive. During this process, the doctor may employ a range of effective strategies, including behavior therapy and exploring innovative approaches to enhance their daily routines.

Discover how a child's ability to follow instructions is carefully assessed by a doctor or other esteemed professionals.

Experience the comprehensive benefits of a thorough medical examination.

Discover the power of knowledge by thoroughly examining personal and family medical histories.

Introducing the all-important school records.

Discover valuable insights by engaging your loved ones, trusted educators, reliable babysitters, and knowledgeable instructors. Simply request their input by inviting them to fill out a questionnaire.

Discover how your symptoms and behaviors stack up against the requirements and ranking scales of ADHD.

Introducing the all-new and improved This revolutionary product is here to change the game and exceed all your expectations Discover the telltale signs of ADHD in teenagers and adults as expert doctors meticulously observe and document the following distinguishing characteristics:

- Experience a newfound focus and attention to detail with our revolutionary solution. Say goodbye to the frustration of overlooking important details when completing tasks.

Introducing the ultimate challenge: staying focused on a single task. Are you ready to conquer the art of concentration?

Introducing our revolutionary product: the ultimate attention booster! Say goodbye to distractions and hello to laser-focused listening. Experience the power of undivided attention like never before!

Discover the power of following instructions and unlock your true potential.

Struggling to keep your chores in order?

Introducing the all-new solution to your organizational woes: the revolutionary tool that will ensure you never misplace a thing or forget a task again. Say goodbye to the frustration of constantly searching for lost items and the stress of missed deadlines. With our innovative system, you'll stay on top of your game and effortlessly keep track of everything that needs to be done. Don't let forgetfulness hold you back any longer - experience the power of ultimate organization today!

Introducing the revolutionary solution to restless sitting - say goodbye to fidgeting and hello to comfort and focus! Experience the ultimate seating experience that keeps you engaged and energized throughout the day.

Experience the thrill of conquering unconventional heights.

The Art of Conversation Mastery!

Introducing the remarkable inability to remain quiet.

Discover the Art of Diagnosing Infants

Discovering if infants meet these requirements can be quite a challenge.

Discover how a mere issue with growth, much like a speech delay, can lead to an unfortunate misdiagnosis of ADHD.

Discover other potential medical conditions that may present similar symptoms, such as brain injury.

Discover the transformative power of overcoming learning or speech challenges.

Introducing a range of sense disorders, including the ever-present challenges of major depression and anxiety.

Introducing a wide range of psychiatric or

neurodevelopmental disorders.

Introducing the revolutionary solution for seizure disorders.

Experience the ultimate solution for all your rest problems.

Introducing: Thyroid Problems - Your Guide to Optimal Health!

Experience the ultimate solution for all your visual and auditory needs.

Discover the importance of seeking professional assessment for preschool children or infants displaying symptoms of ADHD. Unlock the potential of your child's development by seeking guidance from a team of esteemed specialists. Enlist the expertise of a highly skilled speech therapist, a knowledgeable pediatrician, a compassionate psychologist, or a trusted psychiatrist. Together, they will provide comprehensive support and tailored solutions to ensure your child's success. Discover how they can revolutionize the way doctors make accurate diagnoses.

Experience the ultimate in rejuvenation with our exclusive treatment.

Discover a wealth of invaluable guidelines for effectively treating ADHD in children aged four years and older. However, please note that currently there are no specific guidelines available for treating ADHD in toddlers. Stay informed and make informed decisions for your child's well-being.

Discover the expert-recommended options for older children, aged 4-5 years:

Unlock the power of behavioral therapy: Discover the power of effective parenting or teaching by effortlessly navigating through step-by-step instructions and expertly crafted guidelines.

Introducing the revolutionary solution: Medication! Introducing the game-changer for those seeking relief from persistent symptoms! When behavioral therapy falls short, fear not! Our esteemed doctors have a groundbreaking solution up their sleeves. Enter methylphenidate hydrochloride (Ritalin) and its powerful allies - the stimulant drugs. With their unparalleled efficacy, they are here to transform the lives of those battling mild to severe symptoms. Say goodbye to limitations and embrace a life of boundless possibilities!

Experience peace of mind knowing that our dedicated doctor will carefully monitor and adjust the dosage as needed, guaranteeing that your child receives maximum benefits while minimizing any potential side effects from the medication.

Discover the vital importance of recognizing that the U.S. Food and Drug Administration (FDA) has not granted approval for the utilization of this remarkable medication in children under the age of six. This decision is based on a meticulous evaluation of the available evidence, which indicates that further research is needed to establish its safety and efficacy.

Discover the important message from the FDA, emphasizing the potential drawbacks of stimulant drugs, such as the potential to impede a child's growth.

Discover the expert-recommended solution for parents: training and behavior therapy for toddlers, as advised by the prestigious CDC. Introducing behavior therapy, the revolutionary solution that promises to transform the way parents control their child's behavior. Discover the power of this cutting-edge approach that rivals the effectiveness of drugs in toddlers. Say goodbye to the struggles and hello to a new era of parenting success.

Introducing our revolutionary solution that effectively combats the unwanted side-effects often associated with traditional medications.

Discover the transformative power of therapy as our skilled therapist guides your child towards a brighter future. Through personalized sessions, we will empower your child to embrace new, problem-free behaviors and unlock the art of effective self-expression. Witness the incredible growth and development that awaits your child on this remarkable journey.

Discover the key to your child's educational success! As

your little one embarks on their academic journey, it's crucial for parents or caregivers to inquire about the exceptional educational support offered by the institution. Unlock your child's full potential with the right foundation!

Discover the power of Medication!

Discover the shocking truth from 2014 when a CDC official unveiled a written report. Brace yourself as you learn that more than 10,000 adorable toddlers, aged 2-3 years, may have been receiving medication for ADHD through unconventional methods that fail to meet the established guidelines in the U.S. Prepare to be astounded!

Discover the groundbreaking findings of the esteemed Citizens Commission on Human Rights, the leading mental health watchdog. Their extensive research indicates that the prevalence of toddlers receiving treatment for ADHD and other psychological issues in the United States may surpass current estimates.

Discover the shocking truth: not only are 10,000 toddlers

being treated for ADHD, but a staggering 318,997 are also being prescribed powerful anti-anxiety drugs. Uncover the alarming statistics that reveal the extent of this concerning issue.

Discover the incredible impact of 46,102 individuals who are embracing the power of antidepressants.

Discover the incredible impact of antipsychotics on 3,760 individuals.

Introducing a groundbreaking revelation: a recent study has unveiled a startling fact about babies aged one or younger. Brace yourself for this astonishing statistic: a staggering 249,669 innocent little ones are currently being administered antianxiety medications. This eye-opening discovery sheds light on a concerning trend that demands our attention and action.

Discover the transformative power of antidepressants with a staggering 24,406 individuals currently benefiting from their effects. Join the ranks of those finding relief and reclaim your happiness today.

Discover the incredible number of 1,422 individuals who are currently benefiting from the life-changing effects of ADHD medication.

Discover the incredible number of 654 individuals who have chosen the path of wellness by incorporating antipsychotics into their lives.

Discover the startling truth revealed by the figures above - an alarming possibility of overmedication in babies and toddlers.

Introducing a revolutionary approach to addressing the needs of toddlers and babies with ADHD, even in the absence of established guidelines. Discover the expert advice for teenagers, which recommends exploring the potential of behavioral therapy as a first step, before considering the use of medication.

Discover the shocking truth: a staggering 50 percent of toddlers, aged three and under, who are prescribed psychotropic drugs are not receiving proper monitoring for a full 90 days. This alarming study reveals a concerning lack of oversight in the healthcare system.

Don't let your child's well-being be left to chance - demand the attention and care they deserve.

Discover the shocking truth: toddlers and babies potentially taking ADHD drugs for an astonishing six months, all while doctors turn a blind eye to the potential side-effects.

Introducing the groundbreaking recommendation from the esteemed AAP: doctors are urged to carefully weigh the potential risks and benefits of prescribing ADHD medication to toddlers. This pivotal decision holds the power to determine whether to proceed with treatment or to delay analysis, all in the best interest of the child's well-being.

Discover the 10 Fascinating Behaviours that Define a Child with ADHD

Discovering the distinction between a run-of-the-mill, restless 4-year-old and an individual whose hyperactivity hampers their capacity to absorb knowledge has become quite the challenge. Recent research indicates that attention deficit disorders are on the rise, making this differentiation even more complex.

Introducing Attention Deficit Hyperactivity Disorder (ADHD) - the widely recognized mental health disorder that has become increasingly prevalent among preschool-aged children. In fact, it now affects an astonishing one in every eleven school children. Discover the astonishing fact that a staggering 40% of all 4-year-olds struggle with attention. Uncover the hidden challenges faced by these young minds and gain a deeper understanding of this pervasive issue. Discover the crucial importance of parents recognizing the telltale behaviors that serve as clear indicators of the disorder. By doing so, you can ensure that you receive the precise medical diagnosis and treatment that you and your child deserve, as advised by experts.

"Discover the fascinating world of ADHD, a condition with a strong biological foundation that is often recognized as a lifelong journey." "Discover the importance of early observation for ADHD, as it holds a profound impact on learning and educational development," advises Dr. Tag Mahone, esteemed Director of neuropsychology at the renowned Kennedy Krieger Institute in Baltimore.

"Unlock the secrets of the human mind and gain a deeper understanding of the fascinating brain variations that occur in individuals with ADHD. Discover how this knowledge can revolutionize the way we diagnose and support children," exclaimed Mahone with unwavering confidence. Discover the fascinating world of neuroscience! Recent research has unveiled a captivating finding: the caudate nuclei, a brain region, exhibits a smaller size in children diagnosed with ADHD compared to their peers. This intriguing insight sheds light on the intricate workings of the human brain. Experience the power of the region as it takes charge of your skills and cognitive control.

Introducing Mahone's expert advice: Parents, it is highly recommended that you engage in a conversation with your trusted doctor if you happen to observe any of these concerning behaviors in your precious three or four-year-olds:

- Experience the thrill of regular climbing, defying all limits and pushing boundaries, even when instructed otherwise. Embrace the adventure and unleash your inner daredevil.

- Introducing the epitome of perpetual motion - the constant leg shaker! With an inability to sit still and an irresistible urge to squirm, this restless foot is always accompanied by a symphony of regular movements. Prepare to be captivated by the mesmerizing dance of perpetual motion!

- Introducing the Lightning Pace™ - a revolutionary way to move with unparalleled speed and agility. Say goodbye to the risks of walking too quickly and hello to a world of effortless motion. No longer will you have to worry about the dreaded stitches that can result from a lack of caution. With Lightning Pace™, you can confidently navigate your surroundings at lightning speed, knowing that you are protected from harm. Experience the freedom of movement like never before with Lightning Pace™.

- Discover the transformative power of peaceful relationships with others. Say goodbye to aggression and create a harmonious environment for your child to thrive in.

- Introducing the ultimate playmate who knows how to make some noise! With their unmatched volume and energy, they'll bring a whole new level of excitement to playtime.

- Introducing the art of cautiousness and vigilance when encountering unfamiliar individuals.

- Introducing the epitome of fearlessness in the face of danger.

- Introducing the revolutionary solution for those who struggle with maintaining focus: our groundbreaking product eliminates the frustration of losing interest within minutes. Say goodbye to distractions and hello to enhanced concentration!

Introducing a revolutionary approach: Say goodbye to activities that demand your child's attention for longer than a mere minute or two.

C h a p t e r   5

Discover the power of eight effective methods to discipline Unlocking the Potential of Children with ADHD

Discover the unique discipline strategies that can make a world of difference for children with ADHD. Discover the power of a few simple tweaks to your parenting strategies and witness your child's behavior soar to new heights of excellence.

Introducing a unique challenge that some children face - ADHD. These incredible kids may find it difficult to stay seated, accomplish tasks, control their impulses, and adhere to instructions. Discover the incredible power of these self-discipline strategies that can be a game-changer in assisting children with ADHD to effortlessly adhere to the guidelines.

Experience the power of positive attention.

Discover the transformative effects it can have on your

relationships and interactions. Embrace the art of giving positive attention and watch as it brings joy and fulfillment into your life.

Discover the exhilarating journey of parenting a child with ADHD. Experience the boundless energy and unwavering enthusiasm of these little chatterboxes that can sometimes test even the most composed parents.

Introducing the ultimate challenge: finding time to engage with a wildly energetic child. Discover the incredible power of providing positive attention to a child with ADHD. Not only is it a superb investment, but it also has the remarkable ability to reduce attention-seeking behavior. Experience the transformative effects for yourself. Experience the power of effectiveness with our revolutionary solution.

Discover the power of connection, no matter how challenging your child's behavior may be. Carve out precious moments each day to spend with your child. Discover the incredible power of dedicating just half an hour each day to your child. This simple yet highly effective method is guaranteed to reduce behavioral problems like never before.

Unlock the power of effective instructions.

Introducing a solution for children with fleeting attention spans: our specially designed program provides the extra support they need to effortlessly follow instructions. Introducing a revolutionary solution: Say goodbye to missed instructions forever. Our cutting-edge technology ensures that you never miss a beat. Experience the difference today. Discover the multitude of steps you can implement to elevate the firmness of your instructions.

Capture your child's undivided attention before unveiling your instructions. Experience the power of effective communication by simply switching off the television, establishing genuine eye contact, and tenderly placing a comforting hand on your own child's head. Then, with grace and authority, kindly request, "Please, my dear, it's time to tidy up your room."

Introducing a foolproof solution to prevent any forgotten tasks while on the go: steer clear of mundane string commands such as "Put on your socks, clean your room, and dispose of the trash." With our innovative approach, you can bid farewell to the worry of leaving important tasks behind.

Introducing the incredible world of a child with ADHD! Watch in awe as he effortlessly puts on his socks, showcasing his remarkable ability to multitask. But wait, there's more! Witness his boundless creativity as he explores a plethora of captivating activities, all while conveniently avoiding the mundane task of cleaning his room. Brace yourself for a whirlwind of excitement and endless possibilities!

Introducing the foolproof method to ensure crystal-clear communication with your child! Simply provide one instruction at a time, and then, like magic, ask your little one to repeat back what they heard. This failsafe technique guarantees that your child will grasp every detail with absolute precision. Say goodbye to misunderstandings and hello to perfect comprehension!

Recognize and celebrate your child's hard work and

dedication.

Inspire your little one to embrace kindness and shower him with well-deserved recognition. Unlock the potential of children with ADHD through the power of compliments. By recognizing their efforts and achievements, you can inspire them to reach new heights of behavior and performance. Regular appraisals not only boost their self-esteem, but also provide a solid foundation for their personal growth. Embrace the transformative impact of positive reinforcement and watch as these incredible children flourish.

Enhance the impact of your compliment by being specific. Instead of a generic "Nice job," express gratitude for promptly placing your dish in the sink as instructed. Celebrate your little ones for their impeccable ability to follow instructions, engage in peaceful play, and maintain a calm and composed demeanor.

Introducing: The Power of Taking Breaks

Discover the incredible power of taking a break, a truly remarkable method to provide support for children with

ADHD. By allowing them to quiet both their body and mind, this simple act can work wonders. Discover the power of breaks - they don't have to be harsh penalties, but rather a valuable skill that can be applied in various situations.

Discover the power of creating a serene sanctuary for your child to unwind and find solace in moments of overwhelming emotions or frustration. Discover the incredible power within as he masters the art of finding serenity in the midst of intense situations.

Embrace a More Forgiving Approach to Minor Misbehaviors

Discover the fascinating world of children with ADHD, where attention-seeking behavior takes center stage. By showering them with attention, even if it's of a negative nature, we inadvertently fuel the very behaviors we wish to discourage.

Discover the power of overlooking minor misbehaviors, as it sends a clear message that obnoxious acts simply won't yield the desired outcomes. Experience the transformative power of focus and determination as you witness your child's remarkable progress. Tune out the distractions of whining, complaints, and noises, and prepare to be amazed by the undeniable results.

Introducing the Ultimate Reward System!

Introducing reward systems, the ultimate solution to help children with ADHD stay focused and follow instructions flawlessly. With the power to motivate and inspire, these systems work wonders in encouraging kids to showcase their very best behavior. Say goodbye to distractions and hello to success!

Experience the power of allowing natural consequences to shape your life.

By embracing the natural flow of cause and effect, you can unlock a world of growth and self-discovery. Let go of control and let the universe guide you towards the outcomes you truly

Introducing the art of effective discipline for children with ADHD - a skill that requires careful selection of battles. Discover the power of balance in parenting. Instead of constantly criticizing your child and making them feel inadequate, consider allowing some habits to slide. By doing so, not only will you help your child's self-esteem flourish, but you'll also preserve your own sanity.

Discover the power of embracing natural implications, which often prove more effective than trying to persuade a young mind to make wiser choices. Introducing a revolutionary approach: when your little one adamantly refuses to take a break from their playtime to indulge in a nourishing lunch, grant them the freedom to forgo their midday meal. Experience the undeniable truth that hunger will inevitably strike, leaving him with no choice but to endure until the grand feast of supper. Discover the secret to enjoying a prompt and satisfying lunch.

Experience the power of collaboration by working hand in hand with your child's dedicated teacher.

Discover the powerful impact of parent-teacher meetings on your child's academic success. By engaging in open and meaningful conversations with your child's dedicated educator, you can unlock a world of opportunities for your little one to thrive in school. Discover the power of flexibility in assignments for children, granting them the extra time they need to achieve their goals in assessments.

Experience the transformative power of behavioral adjustments. By encouraging a young individual with ADHD to observe recess, we can address and alleviate the compounding behavioral problems. Take action now and witness the positive changes unfold. Discover the essential importance of engaging with your child in order to craft a powerful behavior management plan that will effectively bolster your little one's ability to navigate and control their symptoms.

Introducing a highly effective behavior management plan that is not only useful at home, but also in school. Discover the power of this remarkable solution today!

Unlock a world of possibilities for your child with the thoughtful gifts they receive from their teacher. These special tokens can be exchanged for exciting privileges at home, like indulging in their favorite TV shows or exploring the digital realm on the computer. Give your child the gift of choice and watch their imagination soar!

Chapter 6

Effective Lifestyle Modifications and Natural Treatments for ADHD

Discover the Power of Natural Treatments for ADHD

Introducing the remarkable conditions known as Attention Deficit Hyperactivity Disorder (ADHD) and Attention Deficit Disorder (ADD). These extraordinary neurological and behavior-related conditions can present challenges in the realm of concentration, while also manifesting as impulsiveness and an abundance of energy.

Discover the incredible world of individuals with ADHD symptoms, where concentration becomes a thrilling challenge and sitting still becomes an exhilarating adventure. Discover the remarkable distinction between individuals with ADHD and those with ADD. Experience the captivating world of heightened energy and unparalleled focus that sets some people with ADHD apart from the rest. Unleash the power of their unique abilities and witness the extraordinary impact they can have.

Experience the world of ADHD, a condition that can affect children as young as seven and continue to shape their lives well into adulthood. Discover how this disorder, known for its impact on focus and attention, can persist through the teenage years and beyond. Discover the staggering impact of ADHD on American children and adults. With approximately 9% of children aged 13 to 18 and over 4% of adults affected, this condition demands attention.

Discover the startling truth about the rising number of children diagnosed with ADHD. The renowned National Institute of Mental Health reveals that this alarming trend continues to grow, leaving experts puzzled. Leading doctors and researchers point to crucial factors such as dietary choices, sleep patterns, and even breathing habits as potential contributors to the surge in ADHD cases.

Discover the groundbreaking findings that reveal how insomnia, circadian rhythm disturbances, and sleep-disordered breathing, including jaws breathing, can lead to the emergence of symptoms associated with ADHD.

Discover the groundbreaking findings of researchers who reveal the profound impact of ADHD on psychological well-being, educational attainment, and psychiatric health in the long run. Discover the power of early analysis and treatment to steer clear of the debilitating implications of this condition.

Unveiling the Mysteries: Discovering the Causes of ADD/ADHD

Discover the fascinating findings from numerous international studies that reveal the intricate connection between ADHD and genetics, environment, and dietary choices. These insightful research findings suggest that these factors may potentially heighten the risk of ADHD and even exacerbate its symptoms, as highlighted by esteemed researchers.

Discover the hidden culprits behind ADD/ADHD symptoms: refined sugar, artificial sweeteners, additives, unbalanced meals, preservatives, and even food allergies.

Take control of your health and unlock your true potential.

Discover the telltale signs of ADD/ADHD

Experience the unique range of symptoms that can vary from person to person, influenced by the environment, diet, and a myriad of other factors.

Discover the telltale signs of ADHD/ADD in children

Introducing the all-new, incredibly versatile individual who possesses a remarkable ability to effortlessly adapt to any situation. With a penchant for exploration and a curious mind that knows no bounds, this extraordinary individual may occasionally find

Introducing a personality trait that craves excitement and thrives on constant stimulation: the one who gets bored quickly.

Struggling to stay organized and finish tasks?

Are you tired of constantly misplacing your belongings? Say goodbye to the frustration of losing things with our revolutionary solution.

Introducing a revolutionary product that will change the way you communicate - the "Doesn't Listen" solution. Say goodbye to frustrating conversations and hello to effective communication. With its cutting-edge technology, this product

Introducing a solution to the challenge of difficulty in following instructions.

- Introducing the Fidgety Behavior and Squirming Solution!

- Experience the challenge of finding stillness and embracing silence.

- Experience the thrill of impatience.

Discover the telltale signs of ADD/ADHD that adults may exhibit.

Introducing the ultimate challenge: difficulty concentrating. Whether you're tackling an activity, job, or engaging in a conversation, this elusive foe is here to test your focus. Brace yourself for a battle of attention like no other.

- Experience a newfound sense of tranquility as you bid farewell to psychological and physical restlessness.

- Experience the thrill of regular mood swings!

- Introducing a fiery personality with a penchant for passion and a tendency to unleash their emotions.

- Introducing our revolutionary solution: the antidote to disorganization.

- Discover the incredible power of having a low tolerance for people, situations, and surroundings. Embrace a life where you refuse to settle for anything less than what you truly deserve. Say goodbye to mediocrity and hello to a world where you demand excellence in every aspect of your life.

- Experience the thrill of unpredictable connections.

- Experience the thrill of heightened risk with our

revolutionary product. Prepare to be captivated by the addictive nature of what we have to offer.

Discover the cutting-edge treatment for ADD/ADHD that is revolutionizing lives today. Introducing the powerful medications Ritalin and Adderall, scientifically proven to effectively address attention deficit challenges and transform behavioral issues. Experience the life-changing benefits now. Introducing Ritalin, the remarkable central nervous system stimulant that can provide a boost of energy and focus. While it's important to note that Ritalin may have some potential side effects, such as temporary nervousness, agitation, or insomnia, rest assured that these effects are rare and can be managed with proper care. In rare cases, Ritalin may also cause vomiting, increased heartbeat, increased blood pressure, or even psychosis. However, it's crucial to remember that these occurrences are extremely uncommon. Experience the power of Ritalin and unlock your full potential today!

Discover the incredible power of Adderall, the remarkable amphetamine that captivates with its addictive allure. Experience the undeniable allure of prolonged use, as you unlock a world of limitless possibilities. Experience a range of effects you'd rather avoid, such as tremors, hallucinations, muscle twitches, elevated blood pressure, rapid or irregular heartbeats, and intense mood swings.

Discover the allure of natural treatments for ADHD and bid farewell to those unwanted effects that have been holding you back. Discover the incredible world of natural treatments for ADD/ADHD that not only work wonders but also spare you from the undesirable side effects of prescription drugs. Embrace the good news today!

Discover the Ultimate Selection of the Top Five Supplements for ADHD

Discover the transformative power of fresh foods in your diet while bidding farewell to dangerous foods. Unlock the potential of these five essential supplements, carefully curated to provide natural treatments for ADHD.

Introducing the all-new, revolutionary :

Introducing Fish Gas (Omega-3) - the daily supplement you need to supercharge your health! With a potent dosage of 1,000 milligrams per day, this powerful formula is designed to support your overall well-being. Don't miss out on the incredible benefits of Fish Gas (Omega-3) - make

Discover the incredible benefits of Omega 3 supplements for individuals with ADHD. Unlock the power of EPA/DHA found in seafood oil, essential for optimal brain function and renowned for its anti-inflammatory properties. Experience the transformative effects today! Experience the transformative power of supplementation, as it works wonders in alleviating symptoms and enhancing the learning process.

Introducing B-Complex: The Ultimate Daily Boost (50 milligrams per day)

Discover the secret to helping children with ADHD thrive! Introducing the power of B-vitamins, the essential nutrients that support the formation of serotonin. And when it comes to boosting serotonin levels, Vitamin B6 takes the spotlight. Give your child the natural support they need with B-vitamins!

Introducing the all-new Experience the thrill of a lifetime with our latest innovation. Get ready to be amazed. Introducing our revolutionary Multi-Mineral Product, meticulously formulated to provide you with a powerful blend of essential minerals. Packed with the goodness of zinc, magnesium, and calcium, this exceptional supplement is designed to support your overall well-being. Unlock your body's potential and experience the benefits of these vital minerals with our cutting-edge formula. Elevate your health and vitality with our premium Multi-Mineral Product

Discover the perfect solution for individuals with ADHD - a powerful combination of essential nutrients. Experience the benefits of 500 milligrams of calcium mineral, 250 milligrams of magnesium, and 5 milligrams of double zinc, taken daily. Unlock your potential with this carefully crafted formula. Discover the incredible power of these remarkable substances that work harmoniously to soothe your nervous system. Experience the potential consequences of their insufficiency, which can intensify troubling symptoms.

Introducing the incredible Probiotic, with a staggering 25-50 billion models per day! Experience the power of this remarkable supplement and unlock a world of gut health and vitality. Take control of your well-being and embrace the benefits of Probiotic today!

Discover the remarkable impact of ADHD on digestion. But fear not! Unlock the secret to maintaining optimal intestinal health with a daily dose of wholesome probiotics.

Experience the calming benefits of GABA with our high-quality supplement. Each dose contains 250 milligrams of pure GABA, carefully formulated to support your well-being. Take it twice a day to unlock its full potential. Try our GABA supplement today and discover a new level of tranquil

Discover the calming power of GABA, an incredible amino-acid that can bring tranquility to your life. However, it's always wise to consult with a medical doctor before incorporating GABA into your routine, especially if you are currently taking other medications. Your health and well-being deserve the utmost care and attention.

Introducing an array of exceptional helping supplements:

Discover the captivating power of Rhodiola Rosea, a natural wonder that effortlessly ignites the curiosity of both adults and children alike. Experience heightened sensitivity in your neurological and nervous system with our revolutionary formula. By boosting the production of serotonin and dopamine, essential for effective ADHD control, our product takes your focus to new heights.

Discover the Power of Essential Oils for ADHD

Discover the incredible benefits of essential vetiver oils and cedarwood in boosting focus and providing a soothing experience for children with ADHD. In a groundbreaking report by the esteemed Dr. Terry Friedmann, these natural wonders have been proven to be highly effective. Experience heightened concentration and laser-like focus with the invigorating power of rosemary and peppermint oils. These remarkable oils have been scientifically proven to enhance alertness and elevate memory, allowing you to unlock your full cognitive potential.

Experience the soothing impact of Ylang and lavender, as they work harmoniously to create a sense of tranquility. And let's not forget about the incredible benefits of frankincense, which not only promotes psychological wellness but also enhances cognitive function. Elevate your well-being with these powerful essential oils.

Discover the Ultimate Guide to Boosting Focus: Top Foods for ADHD

Discover the Pure Pleasure of Additive-Free and Unprocessed Foods: Indulge in the exquisite taste and nourishing benefits of fresh, unprocessed foods, free from harmful additives. Discover the hidden culprits lurking in your favorite processed foods: additives. From artificial sweeteners to preservatives and colorings, these sneaky ingredients can wreak havoc on individuals with ADHD.

Discover the Power of B-Vitamins: Elevate your health with foods rich in B-Vitamins. These essential nutrients are known to support a vibrant nervous system, keeping you feeling your best. Revitalize your diet with the perfect balance of organic animal products and an abundance of vibrant green vegetables. Elevate your culinary experience and nourish your body with the finest, naturally-sourced ingredients. Discover the incredible benefits of Vitamin B-6, as highlighted by the prestigious University of Maryland hospital. This essential nutrient plays a vital role in supporting the body's functions and harnesses the power of key brain chemicals such as serotonin, dopamine, and norepinephrine. Unlock the potential of Vitamin B-6 for a healthier mind and body. Discover the remarkable findings of a groundbreaking study that reveals the superiority of B-6 over Ritalin when it comes to enhancing behavior. Unlock the potential of this incredible vitamin by incorporating it into your diet through a variety of delicious options such as wild tuna, bananas, crazy salmon, meats, and other foods rich in B-6. Experience the transformative power of B-6 in improving ADHD symptoms like never before.

Introducing Chicken: The Mighty Protein Powerhouse! Experience the incredible power of serotonin as it effortlessly lulls you into a peaceful slumber, fills your heart with pure joy, and unlocks a world of endless possibilities. Discover the countless wonders that serotonin has to offer and embrace a life filled with blissful moments and boundless happiness. Discover the groundbreaking research from the esteemed faculty at the University of Michigan Health System, revealing that individuals with ADD/ADHD may experience imbalances in serotonin. Discover the incredible power of serotonin in managing impulse control and hostility, two common symptoms associated with ADD/ADHD.

Start Your Day Right: Discover the power of breakfast for individuals with ADHD. By fueling your body in the morning, you can effectively regulate your bloodstream sugars and stabilize hormonal fluctuations. Start your day right with a protein-packed breakfast containing a minimum of 20 grams of pure nourishment. Introducing the irresistible Thin Mint Proteins Smoothie, a tantalizing blend that boasts a remarkable 20 grams of pure protein.

Indulge in this delectable and satisfying concoction that is guaranteed to invigorate your taste buds and provide a nourishing start to your day. Don't miss out on this delightful way to "break the fast."

Introducing our exquisite Wild-Caught Salmon: a true powerhouse of nutrition. Not only is it bursting with the goodness of vitamin B-6, but it also boasts an abundance of omega 3. Indulge in this delectable catch and experience the ultimate blend of health and flavor. Discover the groundbreaking findings from the esteemed Maryland Hospital institution! In a remarkable scientific trial, it was revealed that children with lower levels of omega-3 EFA's experienced significant improvements in learning and behavioral issues, including those associated with ADHD. This compelling evidence highlights the crucial role that omega-3 plays in enhancing cognitive function and addressing behavioral challenges in children. Discover the incredible benefits of incorporating healthy salmons into your diet. Experts recommend indulging in this delicious and nutritious fish at least twice a week. Don't miss out on the opportunity to nourish your body and tantalize your taste buds with the finest salmons available.

Discover the Power of a Balanced Diet: Foods to Steer Clear of for ADHD

Introducing Sugar: The Culprit Behind ADHD Triggers Indulge in a healthier lifestyle by steering clear of refined sugar. Say goodbye to tempting treats like chocolate, desserts, soda, and fruit drinks.

Discover the fascinating connection between gluten and behavior! Many esteemed researchers and concerned parents have noticed a remarkable phenomenon - when children consume gluten, their behavior may take a turn for the worse. This intriguing observation suggests a potential sensitivity to the protein found in wheat. Uncover the secrets behind this intriguing link today! Discover the secret to a healthier lifestyle by steering clear of foods crafted with whole wheat grains, including delectable bread, tantalizing pasta, and even whole wheat grains cereal. Embrace a new, refined approach to your diet and unlock a world of possibilities for your taste buds. Discover a wide range of gluten-free and even grain-free alternatives that will satisfy your cravings.

Introducing our premium selection of milk products! Did you know that most cow milk contains A1, which can potentially trigger a similar reaction as gluten? That's why we recommend avoiding it. Take a step towards a healthier lifestyle with our alternative options! Experience the freedom of a symptom-free life by simply avoiding milk products if severe symptoms arise after consumption. Introducing the incredible benefits of goat's milk! Unlike regular milk, goat's milk is protein-free, making it the perfect choice for those with heightened ADHD. Discover the natural goodness of goat's milk today!

Discover the Secret to a Happier, Healthier Life: Unleash Your Child's Full Potential with our Revolutionary Approach to Food Color and Dyes! Are you concerned about the impact of food dyes and colorings on children with ADHD? Look no further! Our expert advice recommends avoiding all processed foods to ensure your child's well-being. Say goodbye to worries and hello to a brighter future! Discover a world of vibrant hues and captivating shades in every delectable morsel of commercially prepared food. Immerse yourself in the artistry of colorings and dyes that grace these culinary creations. Discover the vibrant world of food dyes, adding a burst of color and excitement to your favorite energy drinks, indulgent chocolates, delightful wedding cake mixes, convenient chewable nutritional supplements, and even your refreshing toothpaste!

Discover the potential benefits of caffeine for managing ADHD symptoms. While certain studies suggest a positive correlation, it's wise to consider reducing or eliminating caffeine from your routine. Keep in mind that further research is needed to validate these findings. Experience the invigorating effects of caffeine, which may include a heightened sense of alertness and a boost of energy. Discover the potential to exacerbate the symptoms of ADD/ADHD with these aggravating factors.

Introducing MSG and HVP: The revolutionary additives that are thought to reduce dopamine levels in both children and adults. Discover the incredible power of dopamine, the key player in the brain's pleasure and reward systems. Discover the key to success for individuals grappling with ADD/ADHD: a harmonious balance of dopamine.

Discover the hidden secret lurking in your favorite foods: nitrites. These sneaky additives can be found in lunchmeat, canned goods, and a variety of processed foods. Uncover the truth about nitrites and take control of your diet today! Discover the astonishing connections between nitrites and a child's growth, type one diabetes, certain types of malignancy, and IBS. Experience a surge in your heart rate, encounter challenges with your breathing, and feel an overwhelming sense of restlessness that intensifies the symptoms of ADHD.

Discover the truth about Artificial Sweeteners: Uncover the hidden dangers they pose to your health and the potential risks they may have on managing ADHD. Don't let these unwanted effects take a toll on your well-being. Discover the fascinating impact of artificial sweeteners on your body. These remarkable substances have the power to create biochemical adjustments that can potentially influence cognitive function and psychological balance. Uncover the hidden secrets behind these sweeteners and their intriguing effects.

Discover the power of Soy: This incredible food allergen has the potential to disrupt hormones that may be linked to ADHD. Unleash the possibilities with Soy!

Introducing the ultimate solution for allergy sufferers: Say goodbye to the top seven allergens that wreak havoc on your health. Our revolutionary formula eliminates soy, wheat, milk, peanuts, tree nuts, eggs, and shellfish, providing you with the freedom to enjoy life without the fear of triggering allergies. Take control of your well-being today! Introducing an innovative solution: Say goodbye to those pesky foods or drinks that pollute the air around you. Eliminate them once and for all! Indulge in a delightful assortment of nature's finest offerings. Treat yourself to the exotic flavors of papaya, avocados, bananas, and kiwis - a perfect choice for those with latex allergies. Experience the aromatic wonders of coriander, caraway, or fennel - all belonging to the same remarkable family. And for the ultimate indulgence, savor the rich and decadent taste of chocolates. Your taste buds will thank you.

Transforming Lives: Embracing a New Lifestyle for Kids with ADHD

Discover the extraordinary power of natural treatment for ADHD and ADD, as parents take on the noble duty of not just finding a solution, but also fostering an environment that ignites their child's creativity and fuels their thirst for knowledge. Introducing a selection of lifestyle changes that have the potential to make a significant impact.

Unleash the Power of Devotion: Empowering children grappling with ADHD by assuring them they are not just another needy child. Discover the power of positive reinforcement! By focusing on addressing positive behaviors, you can create a ripple effect of positivity and minimize negative reactions. Discover innovative methods to foster a deep connection with your child, all while instilling a sense of accountability for their choices. Discover the true extent of ADHD beyond mere symptoms. Prepare to be amazed by the unexpected.

Experience the power of positive reinforcement: A child possesses an innate ability to sense your authentic joy and excitement. Unlock the door to their triumph by providing ample space for their success. Immerse them in the world of artistic expression through captivating activities like painting and sketching. Discover the most prestigious artwork contests in the world, where artistic talent is put to the ultimate test. Experience the thrill of the "quick sketch" competition, where artists are challenged to create breathtaking masterpieces in a mere thirty to forty minutes. Unleash your creativity and showcase your skills in this exhilarating contest. Experience the joy of celebrating your child's unwavering concentration and boundless creativity in moments like these, and countless others.

Unleash the power of regular exercise and ignite the spirit of outdoor games! For children with ADHD, engaging in physical activity not only burns off excess energy but also works wonders in harmonizing those hormones.

Introducing the Ultimate Child-Friendly System: Uncover the perfect technique that caters to your child's needs. Introducing the ultimate productivity solution: a notebook equipped with a comprehensive checklist of daily tasks. With this handy tool, you'll never miss a beat. But that's not all - imagine having a constant reminder right on your wall, keeping you on track and focused. And for those who prefer the digital realm, fear not - our smartphones and tablets are here to save the day, ensuring you stay organized and efficient. Say goodbye to forgetfulness and hello to productivity! Discover the art of mastering task prioritization. From assignments to house chores, exercise to fun activities, empower them with the skills to conquer it all.

Unlock your child's creative potential: Discover the power of nutrition in managing ADD/ADHD. By teaching your child to identify the foods that trigger these conditions and the ones that can provide relief, you can empower them to take control of their own well-being. Experience quality bonding time with your child as you explore thrilling techniques for cooking wild seafood, meat, chicken, fruits, and vegetables. Immerse them in the exciting world of planning and preparation, as well as embracing the delectable eating adjustments suggested above, all of which will undoubtedly enhance their overall well-being.

Unlock the power of restful nights: Discover the groundbreaking findings from Clinical Psychopharmacology and Neuroscience, revealing how establishing healthy sleep patterns can have a profound impact on managing ADHD symptoms. Say goodbye to sleep deprivation and circadian disruptions, and embrace a brighter, more focused future. Discover the astonishing insights from experts on the profound impact of sleeplessness in individuals with ADHD. Prepare to be amazed as we unveil the long-term consequences, such as weight gain, subpar academic performance, and strained parent-child relationships. Brace yourself for a journey into the world of sleep deprivation and its far-reaching effects. Is your child struggling to get a good night's sleep? Are they constantly tossing and turning, unable to find rest? Look no further! We have the perfect solution for you. Introducing natural interventions that will revolutionize your child's sleep routine. Say goodbye to sleepless nights and hello to peaceful dreams with the power of melatonin, light therapy, and sleep techniques. Don't let your child suffer any longer. Try these natural remedies today and watch as their sleep troubles fade away. Introducing the essential element of a well-rounded routine: a meticulously crafted bedtime schedule. This carefully orchestrated plan ensures that you gracefully retire to your cozy sanctuary each night and emerge rejuvenated each morning. Say goodbye to restless nights and groggy mornings, and embrace the harmonious rhythm of a consistent sleep routine.

Discover the secret to a restful night's sleep! Recent research from Japan reveals that individuals who breathe through their nose experience fewer sleep disturbances compared to those who rely on mouth breathing. Say goodbye to sleep problems and embrace the benefits of nasal breathing! Discover the remarkable impact of air load on the human body, specifically how it can influence the brain function of both children and adults.

Experience the incredible benefits of breathing through your nose. By choosing to breathe through your nose, you can reduce the burden on your prefrontal cortex, leading to a sense of relief and improved sleep quality. Say goodbye to chest tightness and hello to a more peaceful night's rest.

Discover the fascinating reason why children choose to inhale through their mouths rather than their noses! Discover the undeniable truth: the key culprit behind mouth breathing is none other than an obstructed nasal airway. Discover the secret to effortless breathing with sinus dilators, the ultimate solution for reducing airflow resistance. Say goodbye to mouth breathing and experience the comfort you deserve. For your little one, our revolutionary nose and mouth mask, known as constant positive air pressure therapy (CPAP), will ensure peaceful nights and optimal respiratory health. Embrace the power of easy breathing today! Discover the power of communication by engaging in a meaningful conversation with your child's doctor about these incredible options.

Transform Your Life with These Powerful Lifestyle Changes for Adults with ADHD

Discover a personalized system that perfectly suits your needs - It's undeniable that everyone has their own unique way of doing things. Discover the ultimate technique perfectly tailored to your needs. Unleash your creativity with the timeless combination of a trusty pen and paper. Unlock the full potential of your productivity with our expert techniques. Say goodbye to missed deadlines and hello to efficient task management. Our specialized approach includes setting automatic reminders, prioritizing duties, and much more. Take control of your schedule and achieve your goals like never before.

Embrace the Power of Technology: Unlock a world of possibilities with the multitude of cutting-edge apps available on smartphones and tablets, designed to enhance your productivity and streamline your daily tasks. Discover the incredible power of these cutting-edge tools that will revolutionize the way you plan and prioritize tasks. Say goodbye to chaos and hello to efficiency with these game-changing solutions. Experience the ultimate focus and productivity with the power of headphones. Say goodbye to physical distractions that hinder your work, whether you're at home or in the office. Elevate your concentration to new heights and unlock your true potential with the help of headphones.

Discover the transformative power of exercise! Not only does regular physical activity sculpt your muscles and strengthen your bones, but it also works wonders in alleviating stress. Embrace the incredible benefits of exercise today! Discover the secret to staying active and motivated with a regular exercise routine that not only captivates your interest, but also brings you immense joy and satisfaction. Discover the exhilarating world of dancing, the empowering art of practicing karate, the thrilling sport of rugby, and the dynamic game of volleyball. These incredible activities not only provide endless entertainment, but also offer a remarkable opportunity to burn calories, harmonize hormones, and alleviate stress. Embrace the power of movement and unlock a healthier, happier you.

Experience the ultimate rest: Cutting-edge research has unveiled a groundbreaking revelation - lack of sleep and disruptions in your circadian rhythm are not just mere inconveniences, but actual telltale signs of ADHD. Embrace the power of a good night's sleep and reclaim your focus and vitality. Introducing the ultimate solution for adults battling insomnia! Discover the power of melatonin-rich foods, cutting-edge supplements, invigorating light therapy, and groundbreaking neurofeedback therapy. Experience the relief you've been longing for while also alleviating those pesky ADHD symptoms. Say goodbye to sleepless nights and hello to a brighter, more focused future! Discover the transformative power of nourishing your body with healthy and well-balanced meals. Combine this with a daily exercise routine and restful sleep to unlock the key to a healthier you. Introducing the ultimate solution for those struggling with sleep problems! Say goodbye to restless nights and hello to a rejuvenating slumber. Transform your sleeping habits with our expert-recommended bedtime practices that guarantee a minimum of seven blissful hours of sleep every single night. It's time to reclaim your nights and wake up refreshed and energized each morning. Don't miss out on this life-changing opportunity!

Discover the ultimate solution to conquering ADD/ADHD with our carefully curated dietary plan, powerful supplements, and expert-recommended lifestyle tips. Discover the remarkable solutions that are not only highly effective for children, but also cater to the needs of adults.

Discover the power of eliminating trigger foods and embracing nourishing meals to effectively manage the challenges of ADD/ADHD. Experience the transformative benefits of a healthy diet for this neurological and behavioral disorder. Experience the transformative power of freeing yourself from the grip of chemicals and processed foods. Embrace the journey of detaching from these harmful substances, knowing that it may take time. But rest assured, the rewards of a healthier, more vibrant life await you. Experience the life-changing benefits of our revolutionary program and say goodbye to ADD/ADHD once and for all!

Acknowledgements

Behold the magnificent triumph of this extraordinary book, a testament to the divine intervention of God Almighty and the unwavering love and support of my cherished Family, devoted Fans, avid Readers, loyal Customers, and dear Friends. Their ceaseless encouragement has paved the way for this resounding success.

www.ingramcontent.com/pod-product-compliance
Lightning Source LLC
Chambersburg PA
CBHW031859200326
41597CB00012B/478